THE SNEEZE

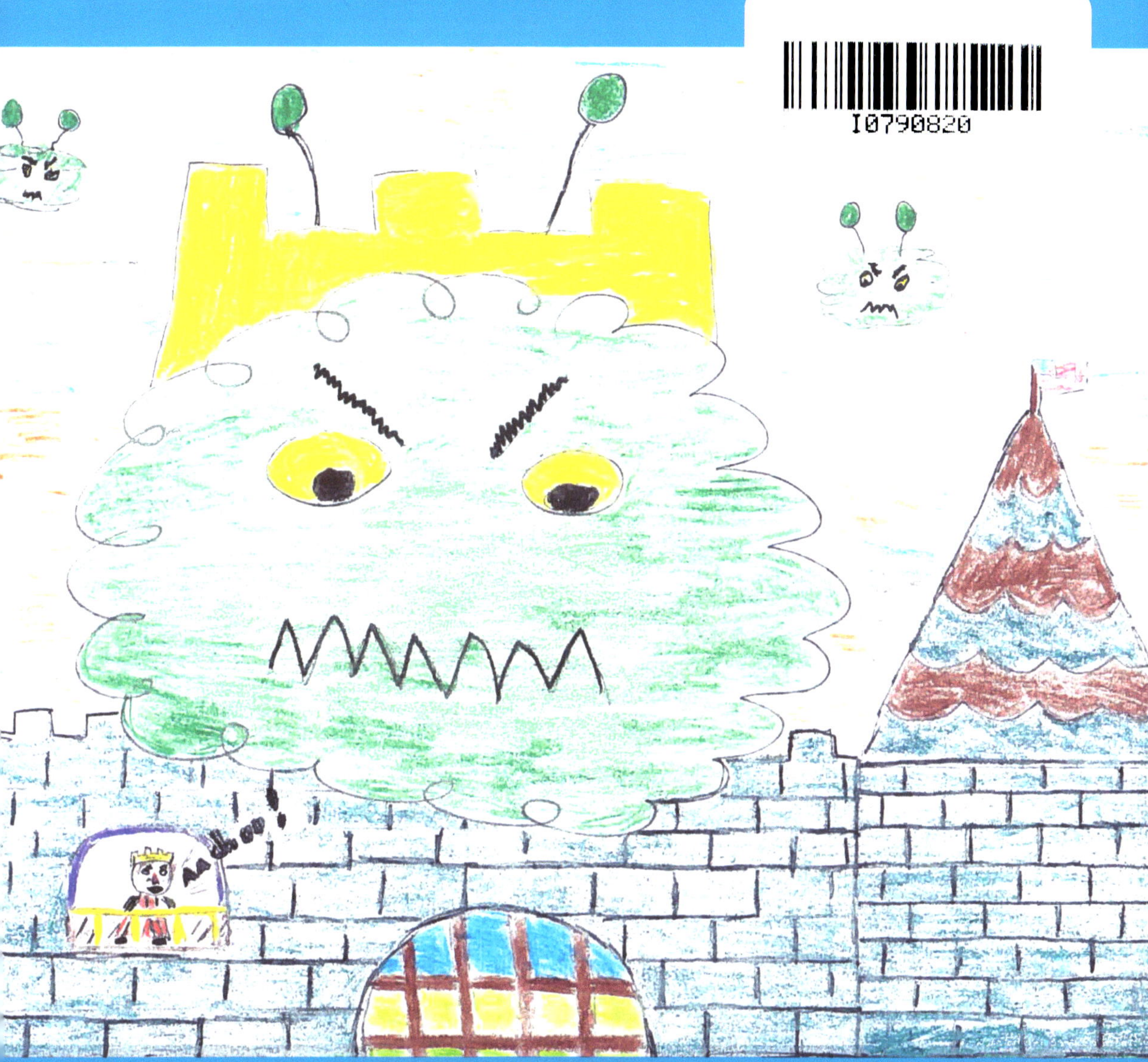

STEPHEN SCARPA PITZ

The Sneeze
All Rights Reserved.
Copyright © 2020 Stephen Scarpa Pitz
v4.0

This is a work of fiction. The events and characters described herein are imaginary and are not intended to refer to specific places or living persons. The opinions expressed in this manuscript are solely the opinions of the author and do not represent the opinions or thoughts of the publisher. The author has represented and warranted full ownership and/or legal right to publish all the materials in this book.

This book may not be reproduced, transmitted, or stored in whole or in part by any means, including graphic, electronic, or mechanical without the express written consent of the publisher except in the case of brief quotations embodied in critical articles and reviews.

Outskirts Press, Inc.
http://www.outskirtspress.com

ISBN: 978-1-9772-2975-5

Cover and Interior Illustrations © 2020 Stephen Scarpa Pitz. All rights reserved - used with permission.

Outskirts Press and the "OP" logo are trademarks belonging to Outskirts Press, Inc.

PRINTED IN THE UNITED STATES OF AMERICA

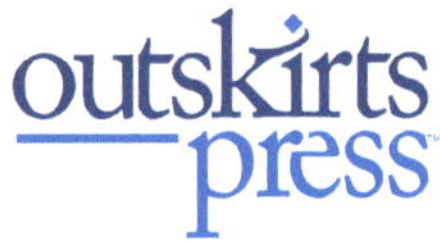

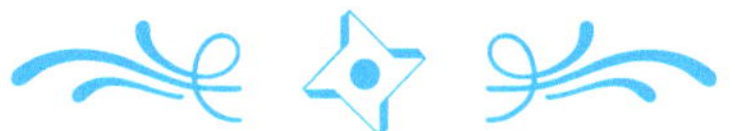

This Book Belongs to:

____

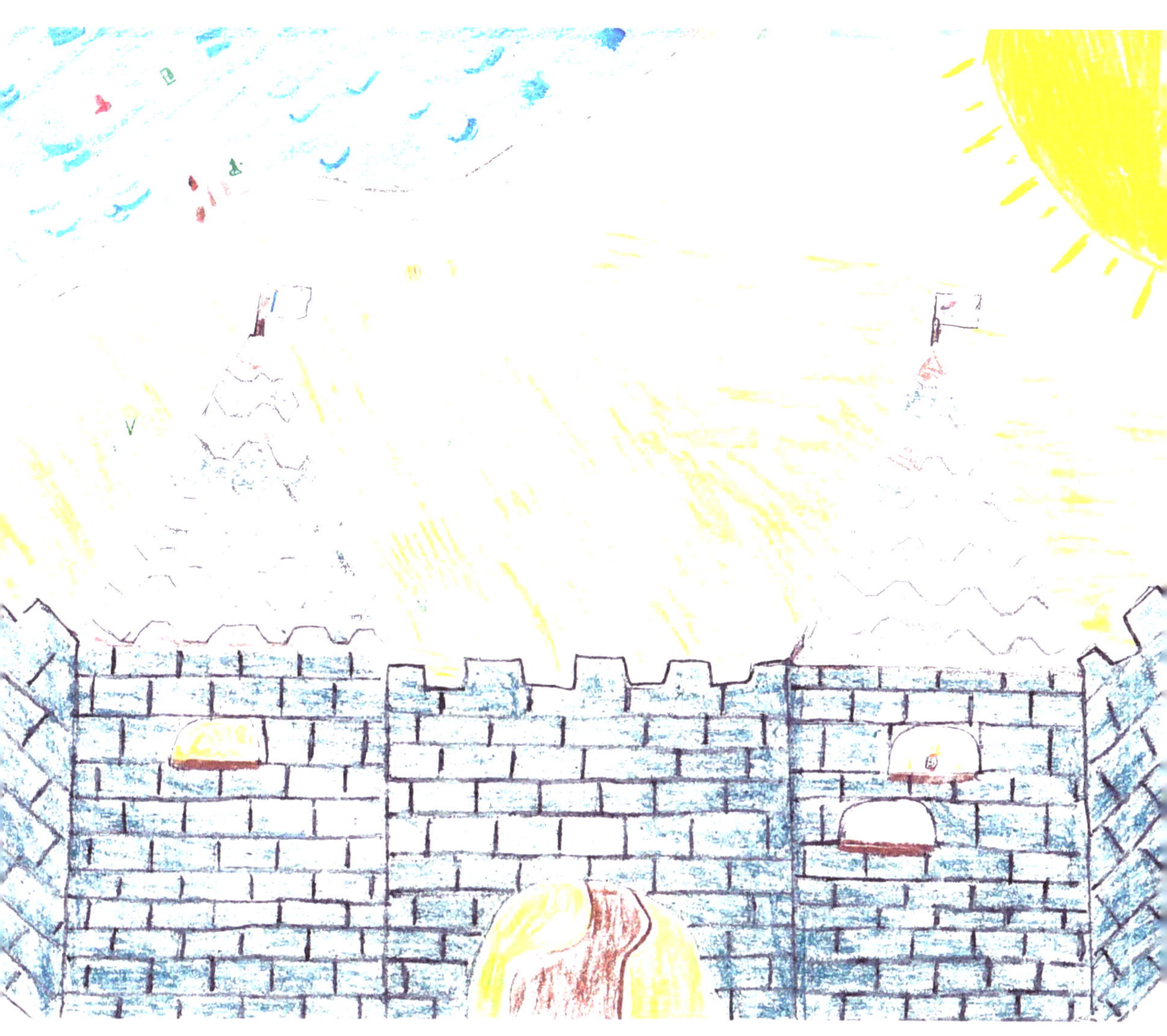

In a kingdom of kingdoms down far by the sea, sat a king on his throne who was ready to sneeze . He had a bad cold, his nose was all red, " If I weren't the king, I'd stay in bed."

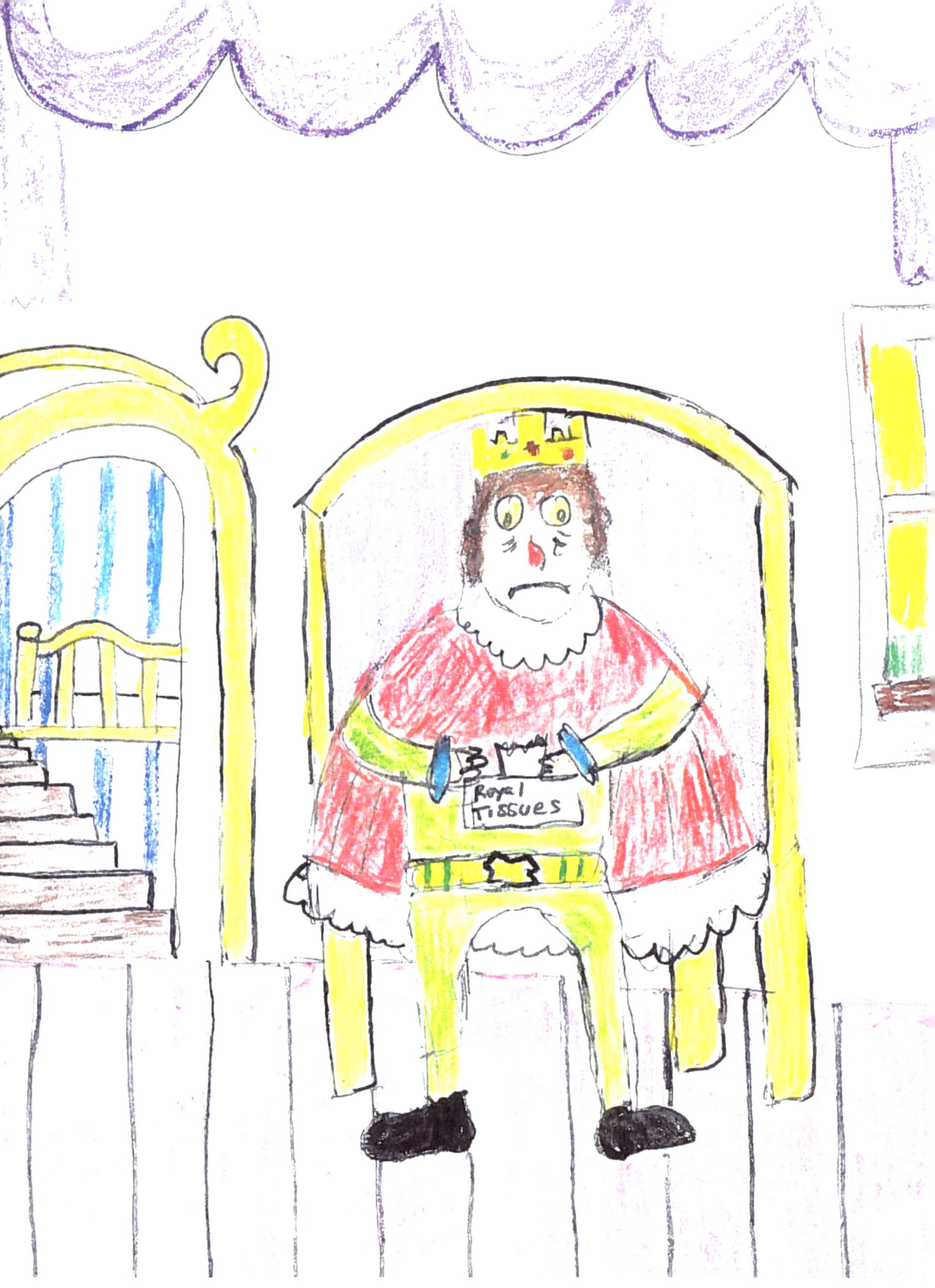

His throat was all sore, royal temperature rise, but the next thing that happened, caught the king by surprise.

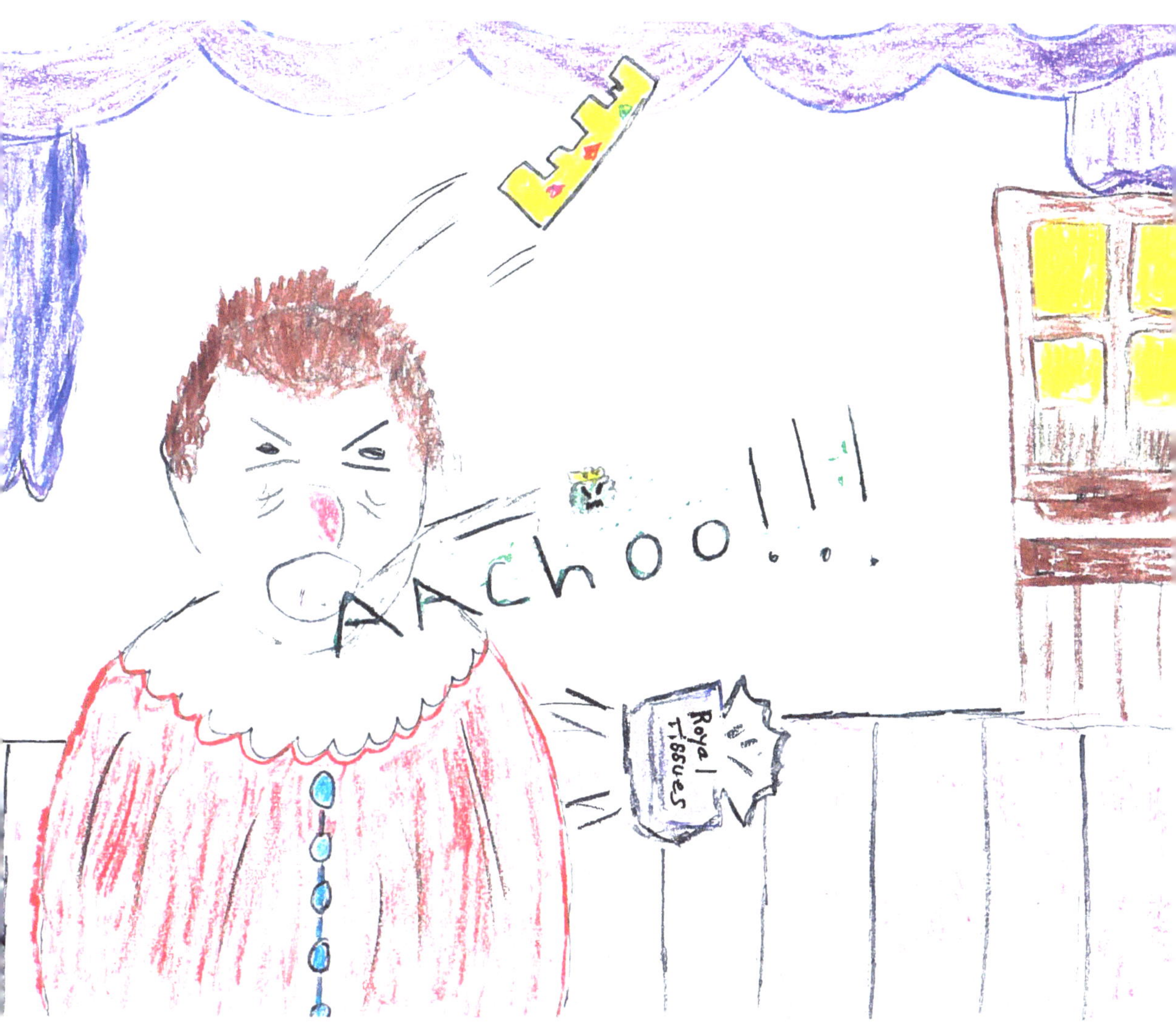

His nose itched real bad and before that was through, the king himself sneezed, a great big "AAAHHH CHOOO!" .

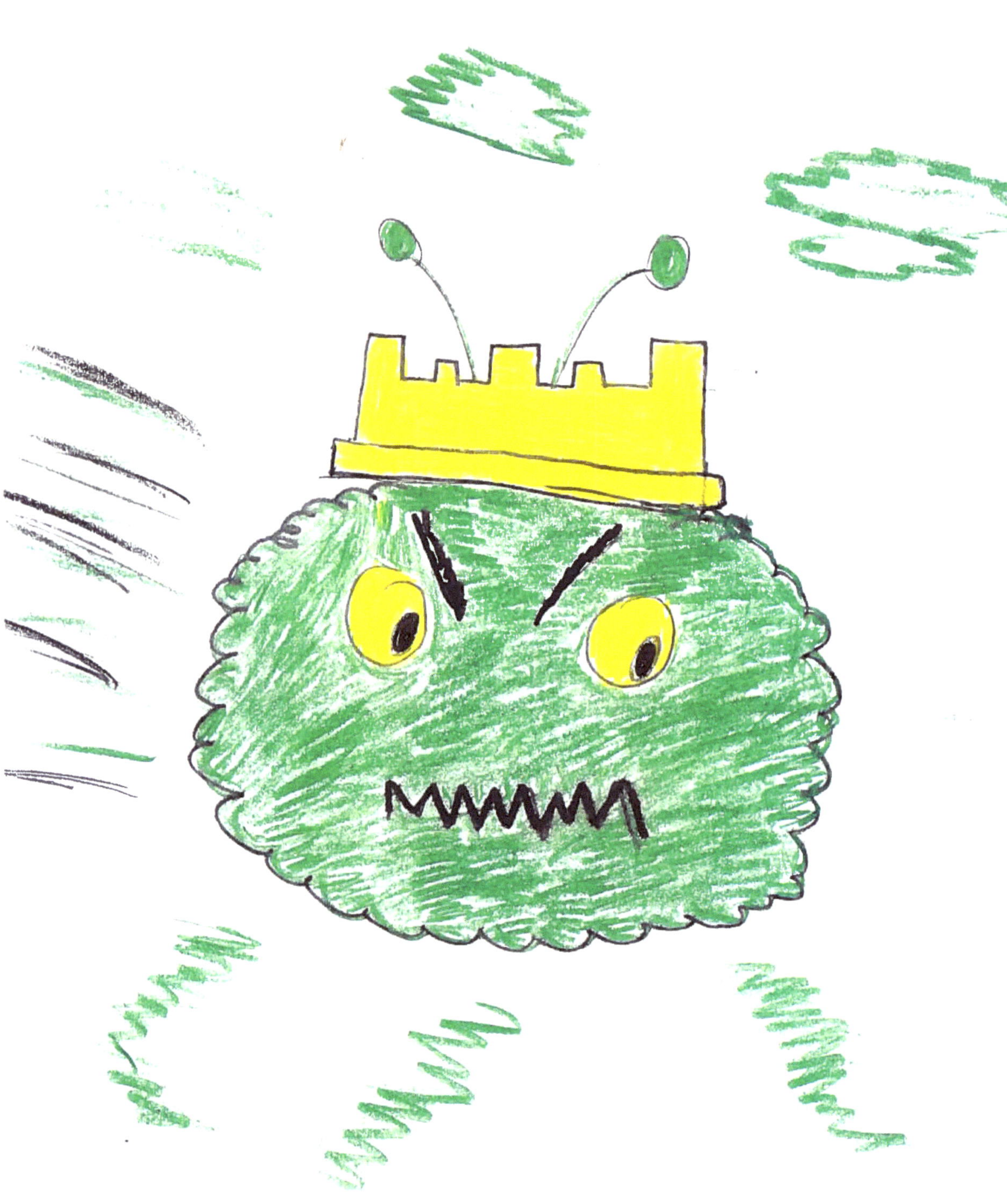

Something flew out of his mouth and blew away in a breeze. A germ had escaped, because the king did not cover his sneeze.

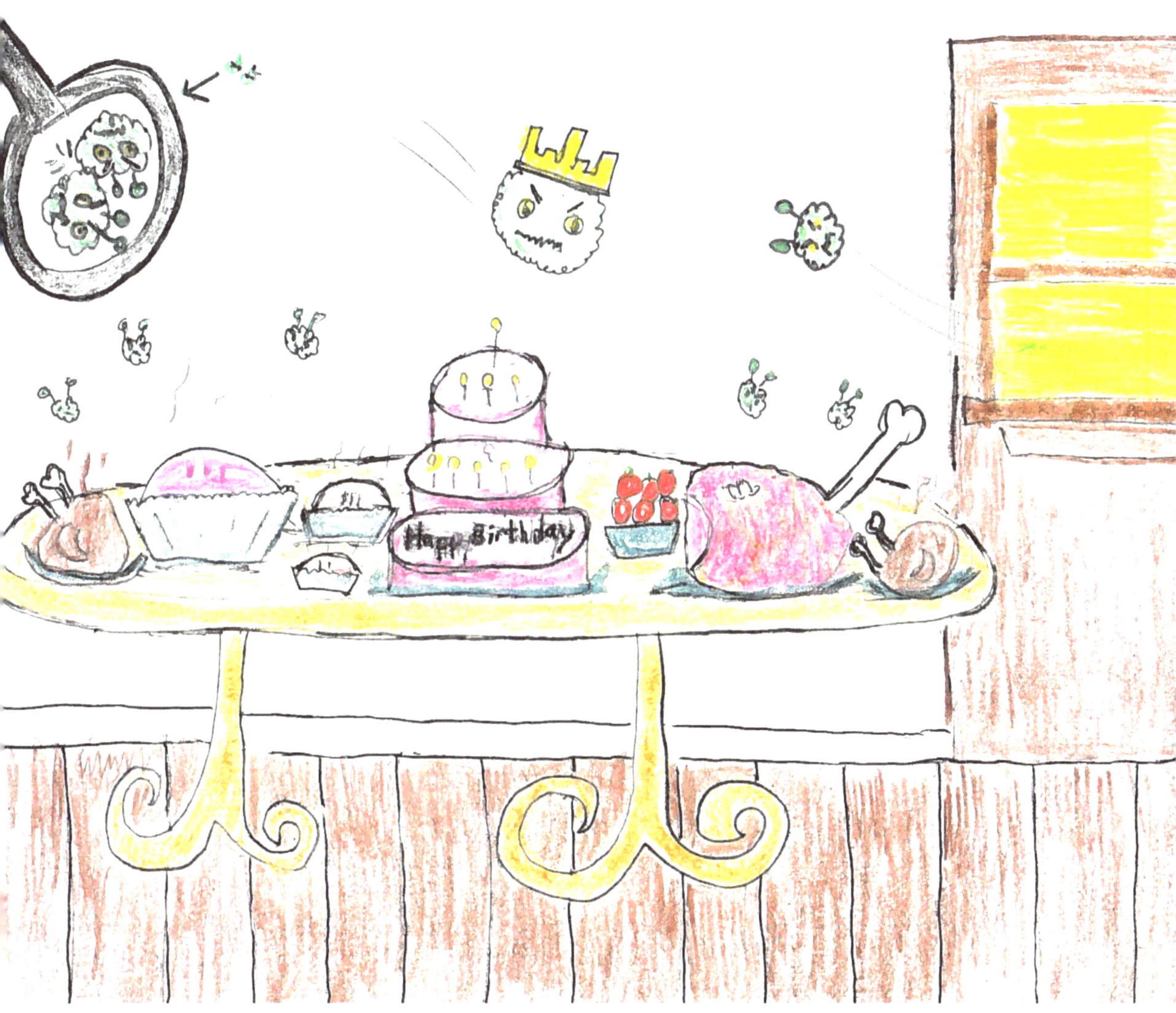

The germ flew out of the window, and through another it soared, into the kitchens, by one open door.

There was food on the table all ready to eat, pastries and pies and the kingdom's best meat. No sooner then landing, on a sweet smelling pie, the germ divided, then multiplied. The food was to be served at the Queen's birthday ball, but the germs invited themselves and infected them all.

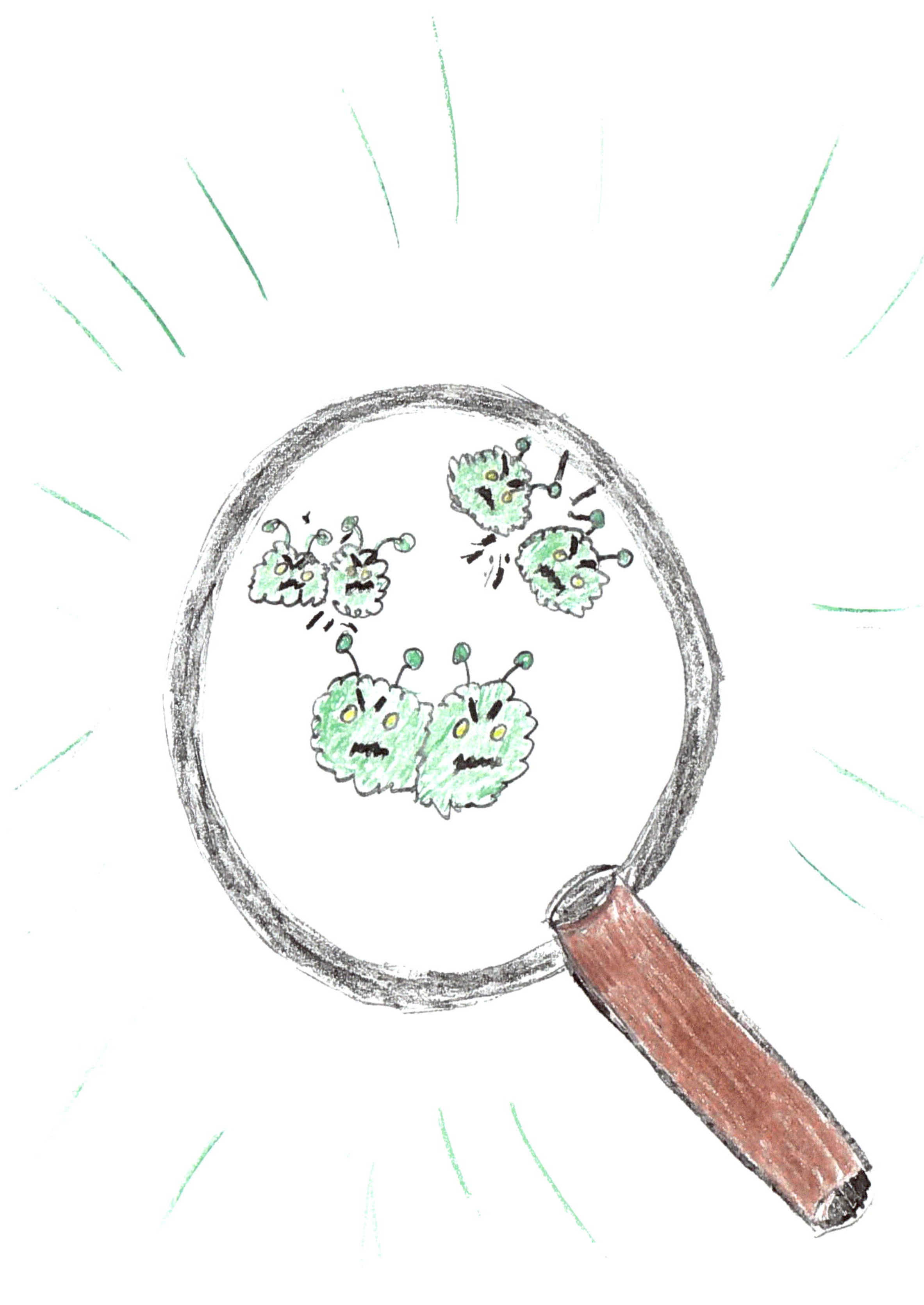

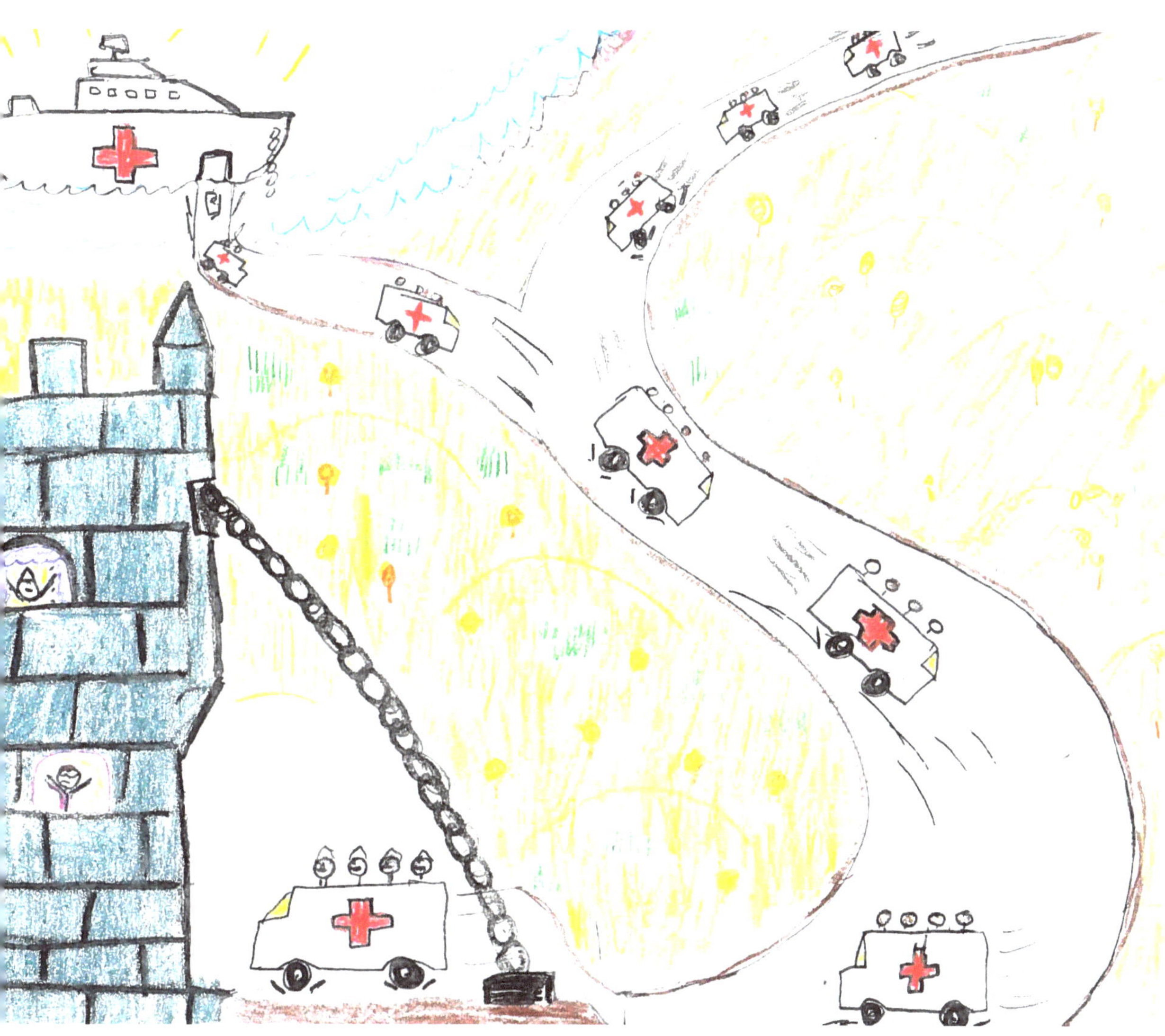

In the time of a fortnight, the Kingdom was sick, so the doctors were summoned and asked to "Come quick!" In came the entire medical team, nurses and medics, with beds that were clean.

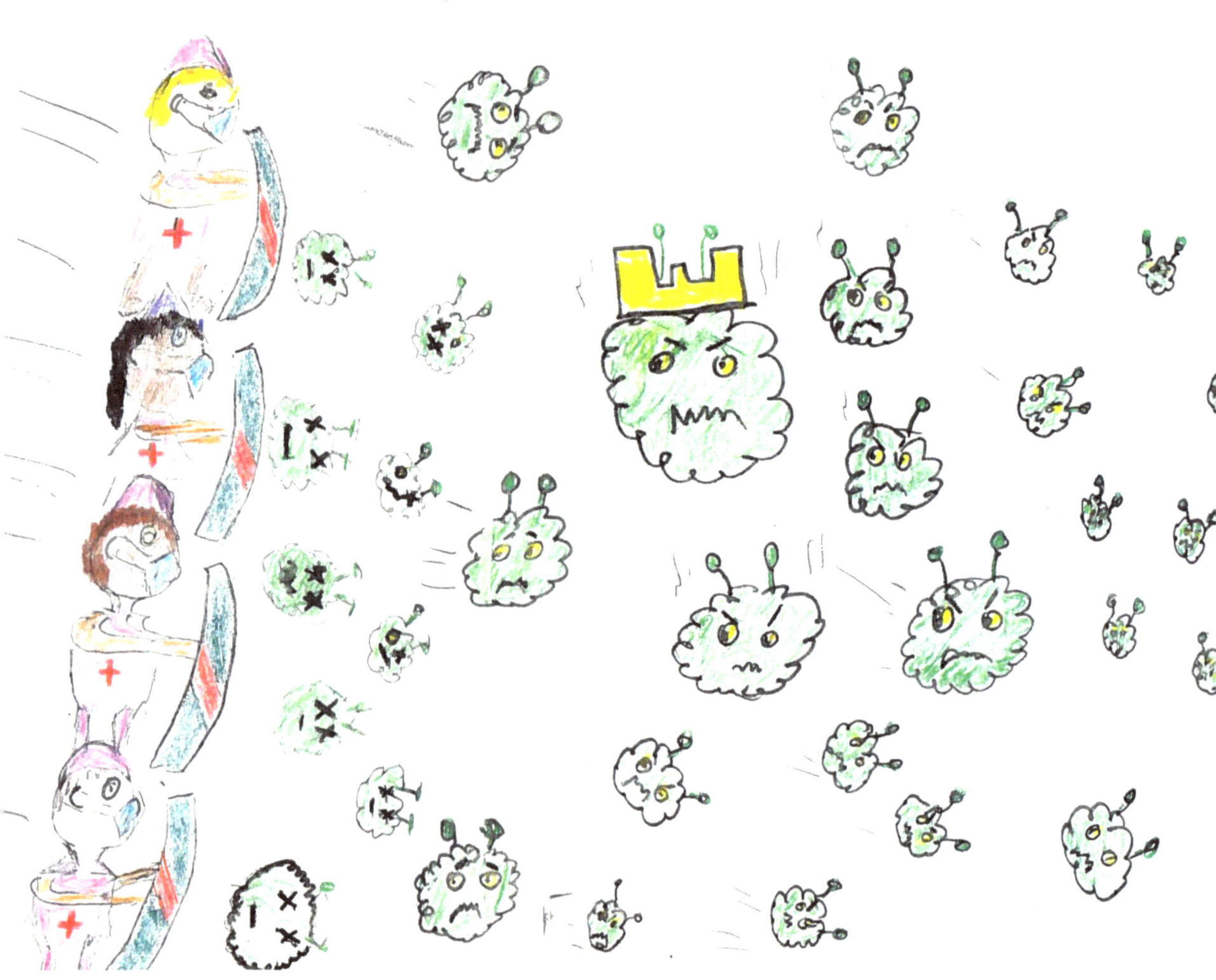

They held the front line with courage and valour, to banish those germs in their final hour.

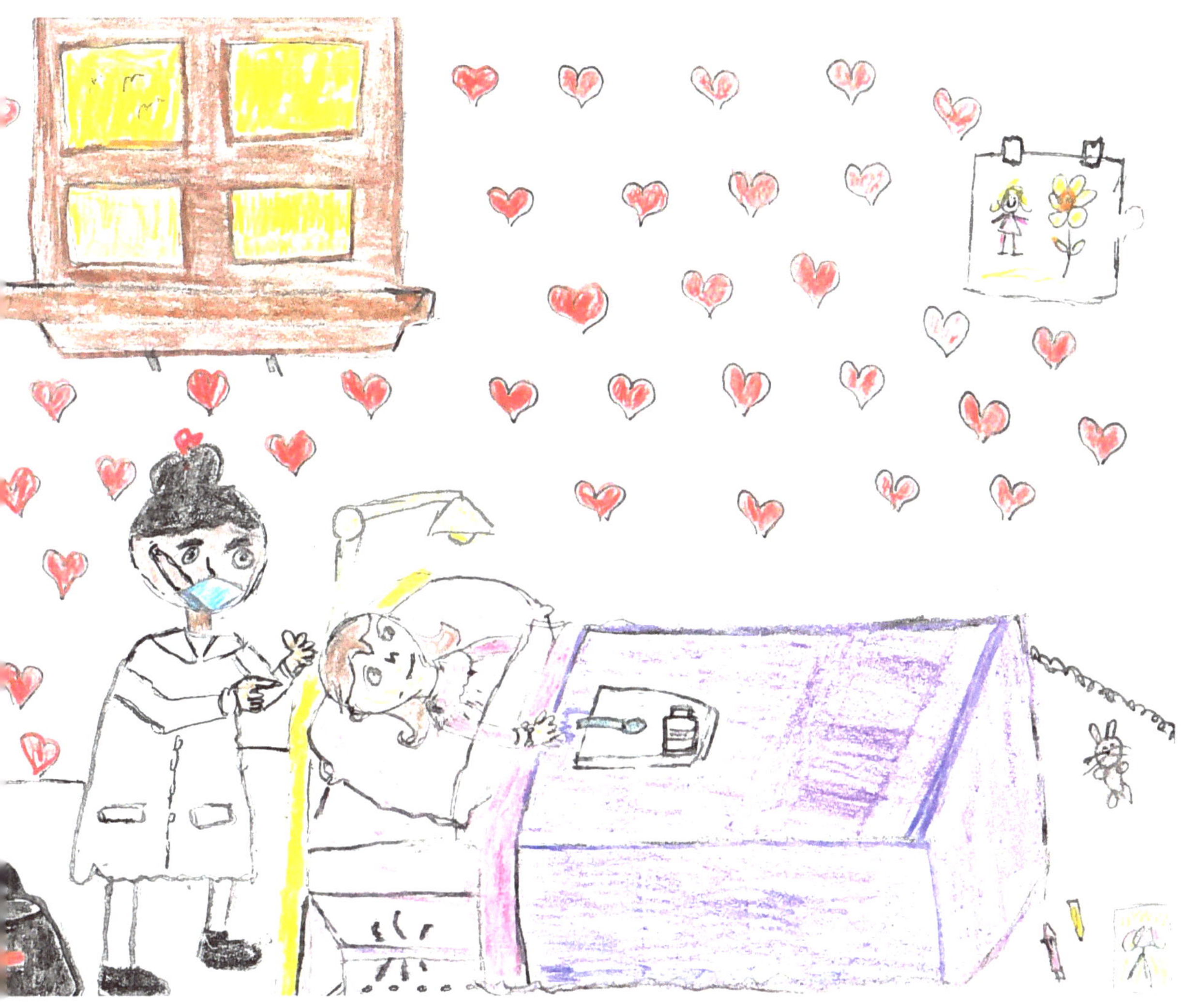

Each patient examined, the same diagnosis was read. "You will all feel real bad for a while, so please just stay in bed." "And cover your mouths when you sneeze", the doctors did say "and don't forget to wash your hands, often each day".

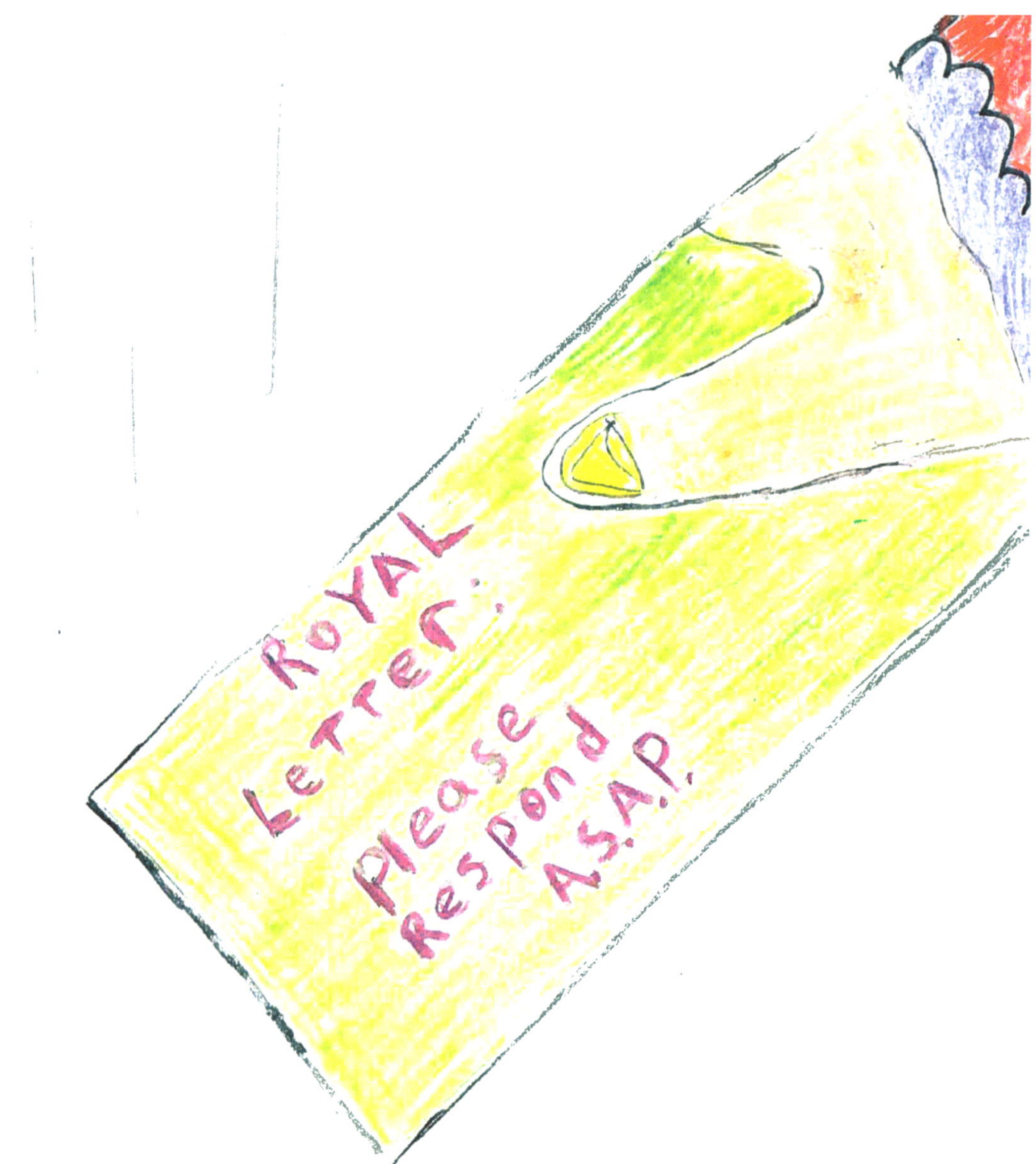

The king and his courtiers all met by letter, they came up with a proclamation while the kingdom got better.

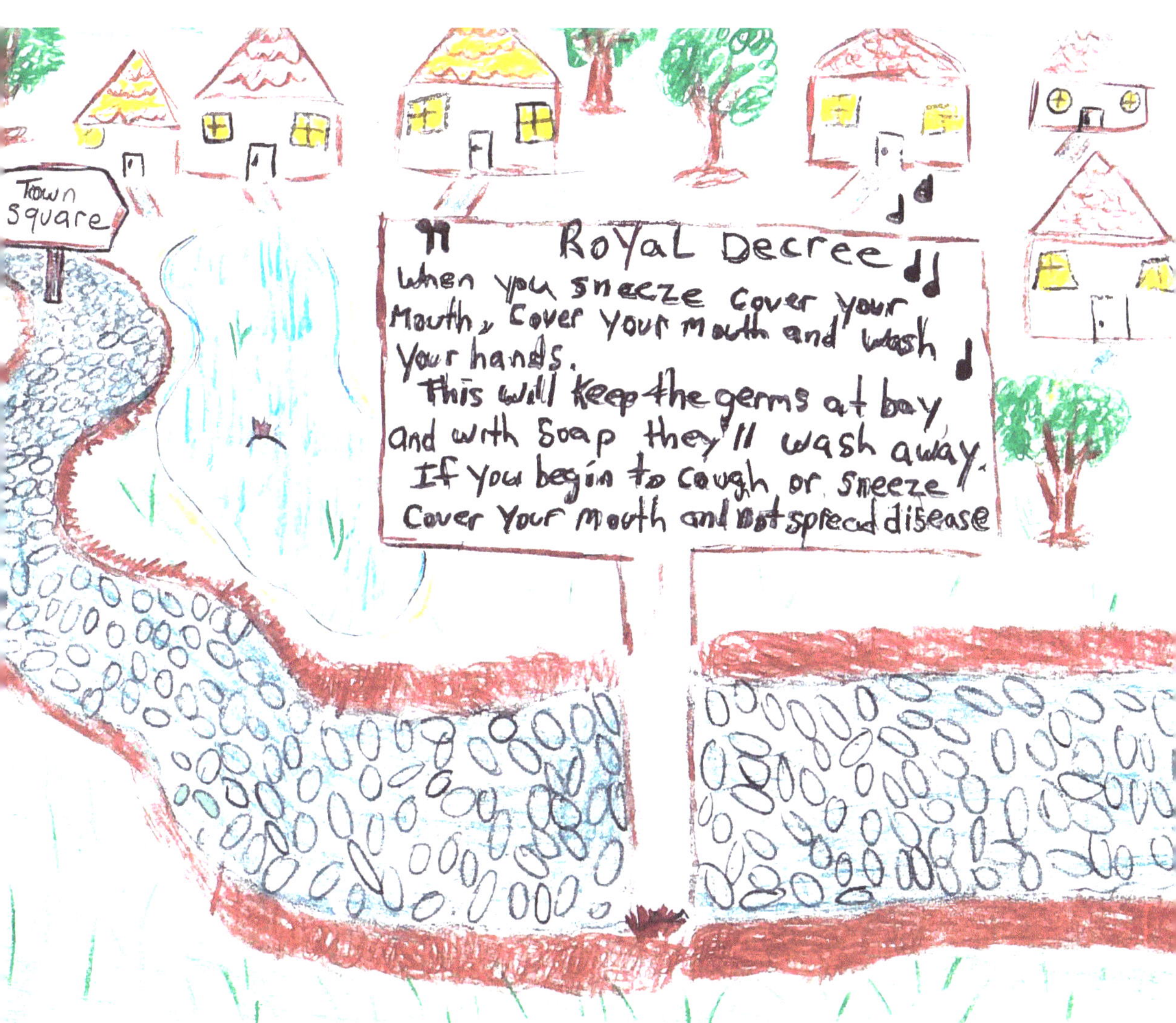

It was displayed in the courtyard, the town square and schools, made into a song, was the old hygiene rule:

"When you sneeze, cover your mouth,
cover your mouth and wash your hands,
When you sneeze cover your, mouth,
cover your mouth and wash your hands,

This will keep the germs at bay and with soap
they'll wash away, If you begin to cough or sneeze,
you should cover your mouth and
not spread disease.

When you sneeze cover your mouth,
When you sneeze cover your mouth,
When you sneeze cover your mouth!

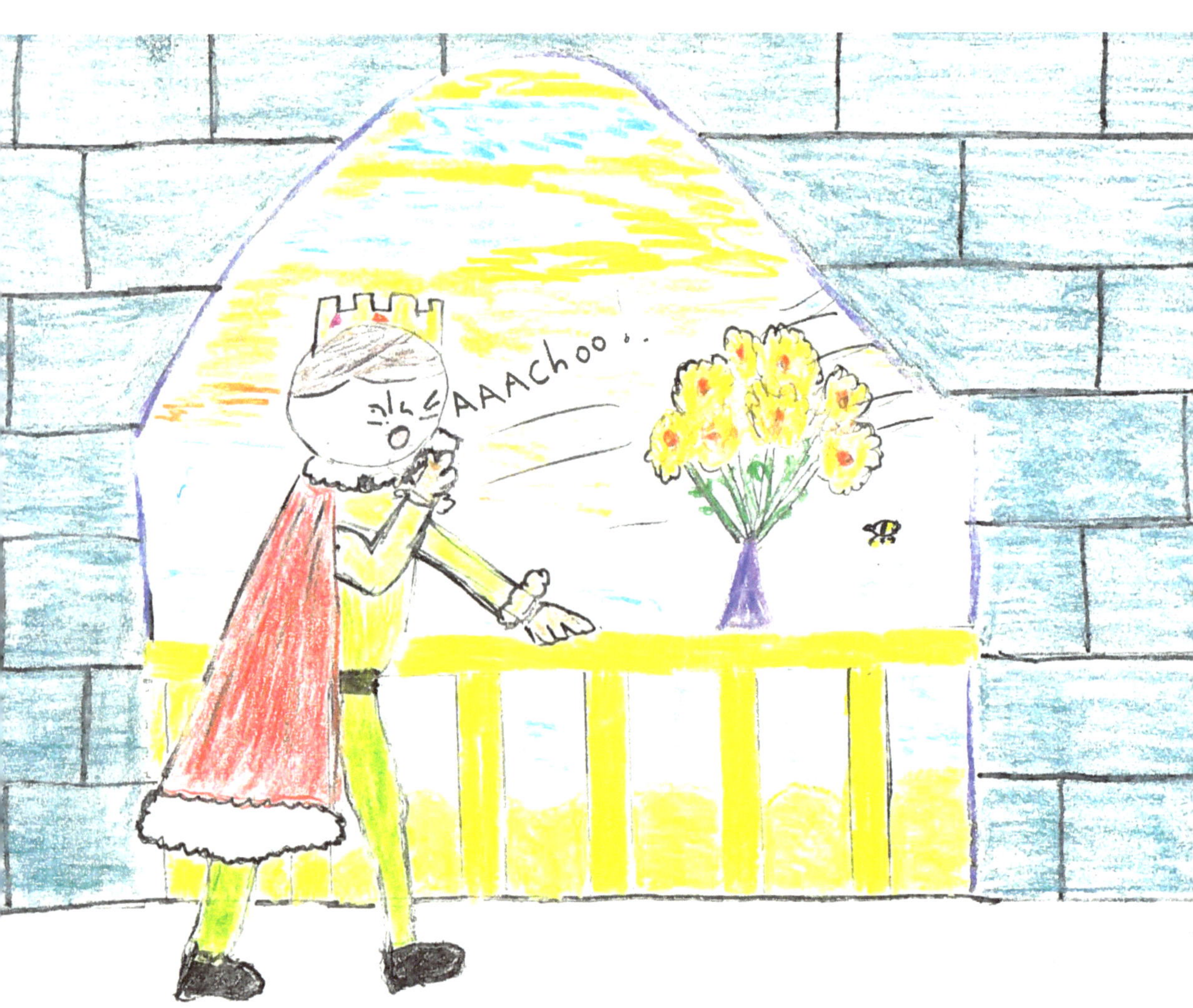

With time brought healing, and at the window he stood, the King looked across his kingdom and saw all was good.

Suddenly, some pollen blew up in a breeze, the King roared,
"AAAHHH CHOOO!"

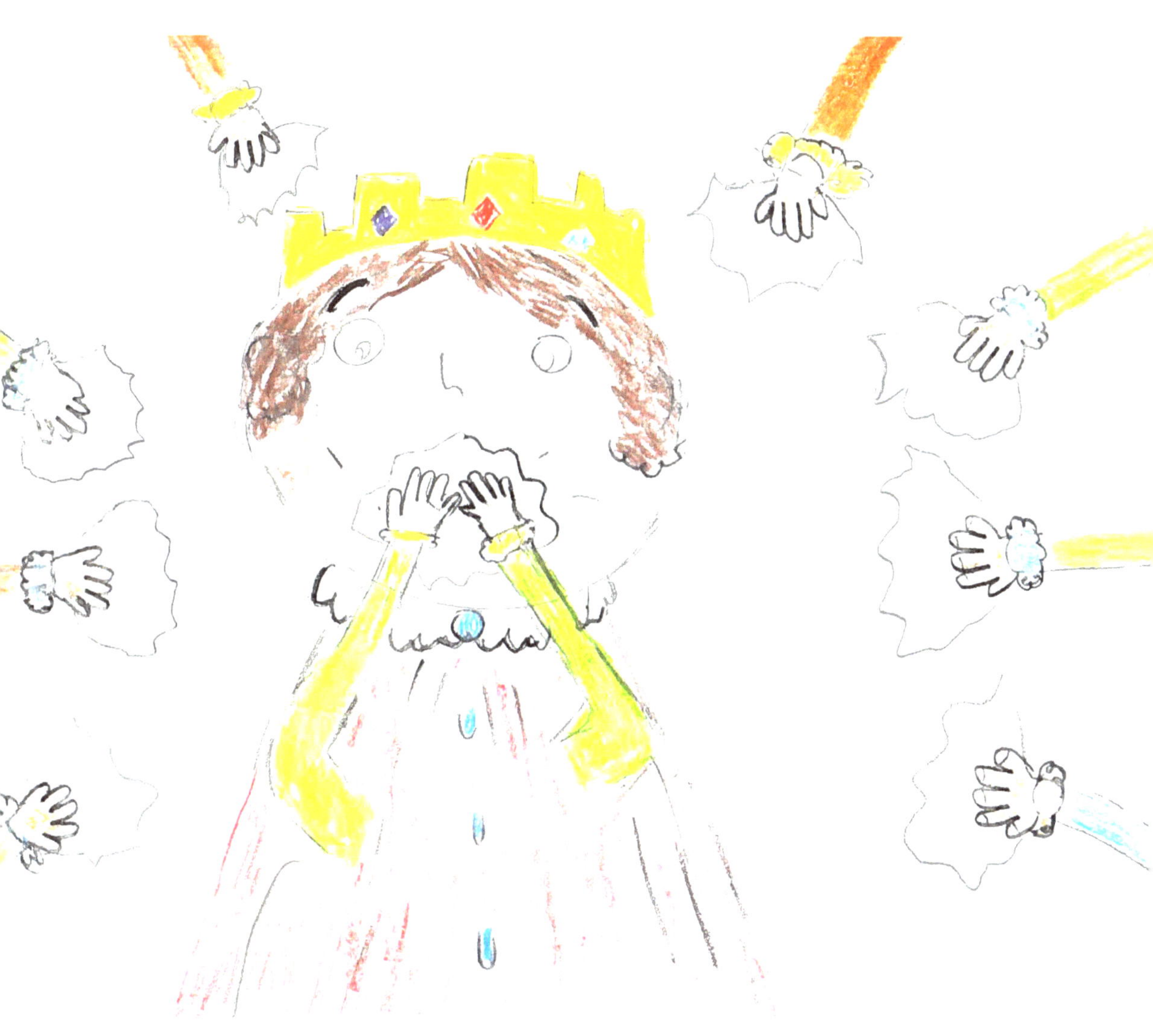

And covered his sneeze.